YOUR KNOWLEDGE HAS VALUE

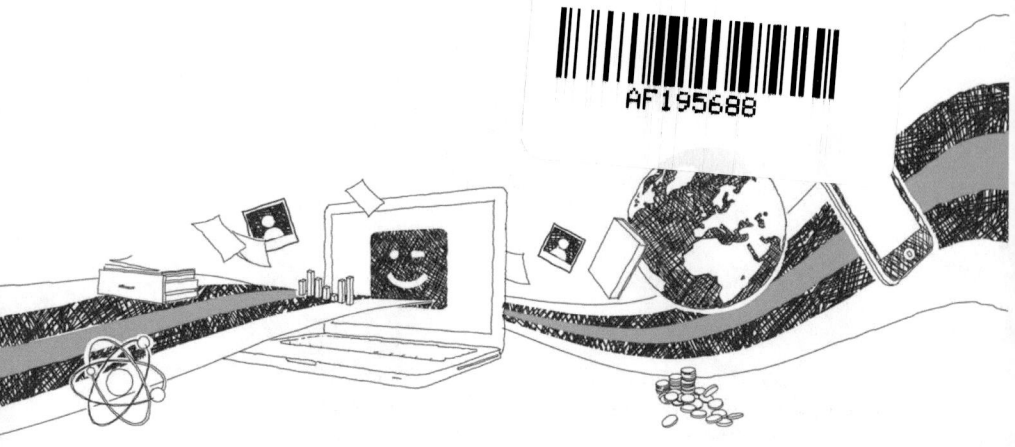

- We will publish your bachelor's and master's thesis, essays and papers

- Your own eBook and book - sold worldwide in all relevant shops

- Earn money with each sale

Upload your text at www.GRIN.com
and publish for free

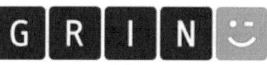

Bibliographic information published by the German National Library:

The German National Library lists this publication in the National Bibliography; detailed bibliographic data are available on the Internet at http://dnb.dnb.de .

This book is copyright material and must not be copied, reproduced, transferred, distributed, leased, licensed or publicly performed or used in any way except as specifically permitted in writing by the publishers, as allowed under the terms and conditions under which it was purchased or as strictly permitted by applicable copyright law. Any unauthorized distribution or use of this text may be a direct infringement of the author s and publisher s rights and those responsible may be liable in law accordingly.

Imprint:

Copyright © 2016 GRIN Verlag, Open Publishing GmbH
Print and binding: Books on Demand GmbH, Norderstedt Germany
ISBN: 9783668353190

This book at GRIN:

http://www.grin.com/en/e-book/345473/studying-brain-structure-and-function-a-way-to-gain-better-understanding

Engin Devekiran

Studying brain structure and function. A way to gain better understanding of social interaction?

GRIN - Your knowledge has value

Since its foundation in 1998, GRIN has specialized in publishing academic texts by students, college teachers and other academics as e-book and printed book. The website www.grin.com is an ideal platform for presenting term papers, final papers, scientific essays, dissertations and specialist books.

Visit us on the internet:

http://www.grin.com/

http://www.facebook.com/grincom

http://www.twitter.com/grin_com

Are we gaining a better understanding of social interaction through studying brain structure and function?

In the following text the above point will be carefully enlightened from different perspectives. After a definition of the research area of social neuroscience, its most prominent method, the functional magnetic resonance imaging – method (fMRI) will be discussed. Subsequently, problems and stumbling blocks in neuroscientific argumentation will be addressed by analyzing two studies using the fMRI method. It will be outlined, why the overoptimistic evaluation of the explanatory potential of neuroscientific results and the relating arrogant attitude of some researchers, feeds the critics. In the next step, a selection of important findings of the last 16 years will be used to prove the importance of social neuroscience for a better understanding of social interaction. This will include examining the structures of the 'social brain' (Kennedy & Adolphs, 2012). Eventually, there will be enough evidences collected to come to a profound evaluation of the claim in the title.

The emergence of the scientific fields of social behaviour and neuroscience is labeled social neuroscience. Its aspiration is to explain the neural processes which underlie social interaction. The notion of social neuroscience was first mentioned in 1992 by Caccioppo and Berntson, stressing the need of interdisciplinary, multilevel analysis for a deeper understanding of social behaviour (Adolphs, 2010). The upcoming of functional magnetic resonance imaging (fMRI) in the early 2000s acted as catalyst for the, by then, fast growing discipline.

What is social neuroscience exactly? Liebermann (2007) defines social neuroscience as the 'study of the processes in the human brain that allow people to understand others, understand themselves, and navigate the social world effectively'. Thus, social neuroscience shares the same goals as the discipline of social psychology. The remarkable difference is the tools used. E.g. social neuroscience works with fMRI, positron emission tomography (PET) or transcranial magnetic stimulation (TMS); tools which allow tempting perspectives on brain function and structure and brought up insights of big importance.

On the other hand, the set of tools of social neuroscience carry huge risks regarding the feasible interpretation of the collected data. These risks, and the disadvantages of the methods used to scan the brain, serve as a fundamental issue in the scientific debate about the range in which social neuroscience can explain social interaction. That is to say, in the end the results are just as good as the methods used and there are certain boundaries to the tools used for brain studies. This is particularly important because the approach of studying behaviour by the use of fMRI to investigate cognitive processes, is threatening the established methods of research areas as social psychology, behavioural economics and even facets of political science (Adolphs, 2010). The aspiration of the fMRI method to replace traditional methods bears the risk of overrating its validity and sometimes results in vastly questionable research designs.

Therefore, in the following we will take a deeper look on the advantages and disadvantages of one of the most frequently used brain study methods. Thereafter, the risk of false inferences of collected data about brain structure and function will be illustrated on the basis of two studies. Studies using MRI-technology make it possible to nearly give a real-time view on the brain. MRI technology measures changes in blood flow, guided by the underlying assumption that an activated brain region requires more oxygen, which is transported through blood. Consequently, a higher blood flow in a specific region is assumed to be correlated with neural activity (Höhl, 2014). That the fMRI method is not measuring brain activity directly, is a common argument for sceptics of the method (Schmundt & Felix, 2012). Nevertheless, the advantages compared to the preceding CT Scan method are substantial: MRI offers a much higher spatial resolution without exposure to radiation as it is non-invasive. Compared to positron emission tomography, the fMRI method offers the opportunity to create event-related designs, which suit much more the demands of psychological experiments. On the negative side, the BOLD signal is not measuring neural activity in a direct way. Furthermore it lacks temporal resolution and does not provide information on causality of findings; a fact, that is often the reason for false conclusions from the data given.

According to that, there is good reason to take a deeper look on a study's methodology, especially in this example: The study, conducted by renowned neuroscientists Iacoboni, Freedman and Kaplan from the University of California, was published in The New York Times with the title 'This Is Your Brain on Politics' (2007). The research team's matter of interest was to examine the way US-citizens feel about the candidates aiming for the presidential office in 2008. Therefore, they asked 20 test persons into the fMRI scanner, where they were shown pictures of the candidates. Thereafter the conductor presented film clips to the test persons, showing the candidates speaking in public. The last trial contained the pictures from the first trial. The test persons were asked to do a before and after comparison (on a scale from 0-10; very unfavourable – very favourable). This more than questionable design resulted in following 'findings': Having seen pictures of Hillary Clinton, participants who evaluated her as unfavourable showed activity in the anterior cingulate gyrus, which is in the judgement of the researchers 'an emotional center of the brain that is aroused when a person feels compelled to act in two different ways but must choose one' (Iacobini et al., 2007). Pictures of Mitt Romney correlated with activity in the amygdale. The interpretation of the research team was that Mitt Romney causes fear in the voters. These are very strong and very specific inferences based on a simple brain scan.

The problem gets even clearer in another newspaper article. A psychologist from Princeton University claimed 'Bikinis Make Men See Women as Objects' (2009), as scans allegedly confirm. The lead researcher Susan Fiske claimed that when men are shown pictures of women in bikinis, the brain region associated with tool use is activated (Dell'Amore, 2009). Both of the studies, which were made publicly accessible to many people, fell into the trap of invalid reverse inference. In case of the latter study, the logic in the argumentation is as follows: if tools activate region XY and women in bikinis activate the same region XY, then men perceive women in bikinis as objects. This sort of argumentation is only acceptable, when the area affected is responsible for only one task. This is the case in the primary visual cortex. For every other brain region it is not acceptable. Thus, it is very important to set experiments in (social) neuroscience in a way that the concerned cognitive process is induced reliably and can be differentiated sufficiently from other cognitive processes (Höhl, 2014). Studies like above are a huge problem for the credibility of neuroscientific results. Laying aside poor designed studies, still, the problem of the mapping between brain structures and psychological processes is one of the big current debates in neuroscience nowadays (Adolphs, 2010). This makes it important to keep in mind that 'no single brain structure maps any central psychological process' (Adolphs, 2010).

Neuroscientific argumentation (especially using brain scans) is very appealing to the public. A study shows that images of brain scans have a vastly convincing influence on the public awareness of research results (McCabe & Castel, 2008). That means that people generally like to believe in what they can actually *see* on a scan. Indeed, brain images are much more accessible to a broader audience than dry evaluation tables. That makes the issue of poor neuroscientific designs even more significant. When it comes to reproducibility and validity of neuroscientific studies, findings paint a rather negative picture. For instance, a meta analysis of studies using the fMRI method estimates that around 10-20% of the brain activations reported in the examined studies are false positives (Wager, Lindquist & Kaplan, 2007). In another study, repeated fMRI measurements lead showed an overlap of only 30% in areas activated (Schmundt & Felix, 2012). Compensatively it must be said that this is not solely a problem related to the use of fMRI. Psychological studies in general have a massive problem with reproducibility due to the infamous 'p-hacking'-practice, in order to raise the chances of the paper to be published. In a big reproducibility analysis, more than half of the examined studies (all from the year 2008) were not reproducible (Arts et al., 2016), regardless of the methods used. But related to the hype that the upcoming of brain scans caused, it is justified to question if the hustle was appropriate.

It can be clearly said that inadequate neuroscientific argumentation, the boundaries of the methodology and knowledge about the power of brain images on public awareness raise skepticism towards new findings and it is true that there are studies that do not improve our understanding of social interaction. But besides a careful eye on a study's methodology and argumentation, can it really be said that studying brain structure and function is mostly irrelevant for a better understanding of social interaction?

A central point of critics on social neuroscience concerns neural plasticity. Critics argue that neuroscientists search for clearly definable regions for complex cognitive functions, although the brain's plasticity is flexible enough to compensate for the dysfunction of even large regions (Schmundt & Felix, 2012). But most of the critics would not go so far to say that the neuroscientific perspective would be useless. What issues them more, is the arrogance of some brain researchers, who carry the explanatory potential of fMRI outcomes and their impact way too far (Schmundt & Felix, 2012). That is to say, the pessimistic position on neuroscientific findings is not least based on the grandiose promises some neuroscientists made in the early 2000s.

Some neuroscientists' overestimation of the explanatory power of their methods raised a sort of sobering when evaluating what goals have really been realized over the years. This gets clearer, when taking a look at an article called *Das Manifest*, which was written by eleven neuroscientists and published in a German journal for Psychology and Neuroscience in 2004 (Elger et al., 2004). In this article the renowned experts analyzed the current state of neuroscience and gave a very optimistic future outlook on the field of neuroscience in ten years. The experts argued that there is progressing understanding on the level of molecular neuroscience and cognitive neuroscience, but the intermediate level, the level of the interaction of neural networks is largely unexplored (Elger et al., 2004). They predicted that in ten years there will be new knowledge about how neural circuits code, evaluate, store and read neural information. Following the authors, through this development there will be huge progressions made in the field of psychotropic drugs and it will even be possible to predict psychic anomalies and problematic development in the human brain. Revisiting the article ten years later the results are disappointing: There have been methodical developments but still there is a huge lack of knowledge about the connection of neural levels. Prediction of individual behaviour is unrealistic at the moment and there are no sensational innovations on the field of psychotropic drugs and still the root for many neurodegenerative and psychiatric illnesses are not completely enlightened. All in all, the major progressions in the field of neuroscience have been made in the technical area and the authors had to admit that they overestimated the explanatory potential of neuroscience (Höhl, 2014).

One can say that the detailed understanding in all categories of (social) neuroscience increased. Of course it is important to go into detail to understand complex processes. But the brain is such a complex system that going into detail is not enough. Adolphs (2010) claims that the realization that no structure in the brain operates in isolation, poses a difficult conceptual challenge to the field of social neuroscience. According to him, a 'full understanding of social information processing needs to acknowledge that the processing is not only spatially distributed but also temporally dispersed' (2010, p.9). That is to say, that concentrating the focus on a single region does not satisfy the demands of a holistic understanding of a complex phenomenon. Imaging methods in brain studies are not adequate to give simple answers on complex questions. Going back to reverse inference, this is rooted in the fact that a stimulus activates more than one region. What social neuroscience needs to meet the high expectations it sets itself is both a detailed and a holistic view on brain structure and functioning. This will go hand in hand with the development of new methods to analyze the brain, e.g. as the use of super-computers in the Human Brain Project for simulating neural information processing (Human Brain Project, 2016).

Having investigated the reasons for a rather pessimistic view on social neuroscience and its explanatory capabilities, we will shift to a different perspective: Why do we even need the neuroscientific perspective? Is 'the social' visible in the brain what are the benefits of investigating brain structure and function in order to understand social interaction?

Answering the first question is rather simple: As social neuroscience deals with complex (not only) cognitive processes, it is mandatory to take a look at the different levels and degrees of resolution of them. To illustrate this, let us assume a research team wants to examine stereotype thinking. Depending on their academic background they will either design a reaction time task if they are social psychologists, or they will take a look at genetic correlates for stereotyping, if they are geneticists and if the team consists of neuroscientists, they will most likely conduct a fMRI study to find corresponding correlates in the brain. Whether social psychologist, geneticist or neuroscientist, all of them examine one part of the big construct stereotype. That infers that in a broader context only interdisciplinary multi-level analyses can solve the puzzle of social interaction. The neuroscientific perspective is of big importance because all mental processes are anchored in the complex system brain. Therefore, it is out of question if studying brain structure and function improves the understanding of social interaction.

The second question is, if we do have structures in the brain that indicate that a social brain is existent. Social information processing can be broadly divided into the stages of social perception, social cognition and social regulation (Adolphs, 2010). For every stage, there is immense evidence of structures that are linked to social interaction. On the level of social perception, there are regions and systems, which are neuroanatomically specialized for perceiving social activity. For instance, there is evidence that pleasant touch sensations begin with neural coding, transmitting affective features of social touch through labeled-line pathways from the skin to higher cognitive regions as insular cortex (Löken, Wessberg, Morrison, McGlone & Olausson, 2009). That is to say that already in a very early stage of information processing, special transduction channels for social communication are existent (Adolphs, 2010).

Social cognition describes conscious and unconscious psychic processes underlying social behaviour. This includes inter alia: perception of other humans (e.g. faces), thinking about intentions, Theory of Mind (processing of comprehending other people's thoughts and beliefs), social motivation (e.g. sharing joys) and decision making (Höhl, 2014). For all those things listed, there is a network of structures involved that is activated when we think of social aspects as opposed to non-social cognition. For instance, there is evidence for distinct neural systems serving for person and object knowledge (Mitchell, Heatherton & Macrae, 2002). Kennedy and Adolphs (2012) outlined the key structures of the social brain. These include the amygdale the insula, the anterior cingular cortex (ACC), the temporo-parietal junction, the dorsal medial prefrontal cortex (dMPFC), the superior temporal sulcus/gyrus (STS/STG), the fusiform face area (FFA; located in the right superior temporal gyrus) and the ventral medial prefrontal cortex (vMPFC) also known as the orbitofrontal cortex (Kennedy & Adolphs,

2012). Lesions in these areas have very specific consequences. For instance, a lesion in the insula leads to a deficit in empathy, whereas a lesion in the FFA entails face agnosia (Kennedy & Adolphs, 2012). The structures of the social brain can be divided into specific sub-networks: There is the amygdale network, the mentalizing network, the empathy network (consisting of insula and ACC) and the mirror/simulation/action-perception network (Kennedy & Adolphs, 2012).

There are exciting and enlightening findings on each network; therefore, a more detailed look into them is of worth. In the following, important studies will be used to highlight the implications the findings have for understanding social interaction in general and for research areas as economy, psychology, anthropology and biology. To start with and in reference to the previous stereotype example, a closer examination of the mentalizing network verifies there is evidence that the vMPFC is active when we think about ourselves and about similar others, whereas the dMPFC is active when we think about dissimilar others (Mitchell, 2006). That is to say, confrontation with people having a dissimilar cultural background can launch cognitive processing in a distinct area. This has interesting implications for stereotype research.

Social regulation is the third broad stage of social information processing (Adolphs, 2010). It plays an important role in human social interaction through our ability to step back and control our thinking and behaviour, using metacognition (Adolphs, 2010). Social regulation is strongly interwoven with emotional regulation. Even further, from an evolutionary point of view one can argue that the complex social environment of humans has boosted the development of more finely differentiated emotions than the states of hunger and thirst (Adolphs, 2010), which we don't even consider as emotions. Coming back to the networks of the social brain, the amygdale network and the affective pain network are of great significance.

The evaluation of the amygdale network's function has slightly changed over the last years. Öhmann and Mineka (2001) examined the amygdale and postulated that the amygdale is purely a fear module, as it evaluates (potential) threats. They underpinned their statement with an examination that electric stimulation of the amygdale leads to fear behaviour (both humans and animals) and that a lesion of the amygdale leads to fearlessness (animal study). Perceiving the amygdale as a fear module is right and plausible, but it is more complex than that. Kensinger and Schacter (2006) examined the processing of emotional pictures and words and looked at effects of valence and arousal. Their findings show that the amygdale is not a mere fear module as postulated by Öhmann and Mineka in 2001, as the fMRI scans show activation of the amygdale for positive stimuli as well, but in a lower intensity. Thus, one can argue that the amygdale has a boosting function for emotions, regardless their valence. The activation for stimuli with negative valence might be higher because of a negativity bias for negative emotions, as these create higher arousal (Höhl, 2014).

Furthermore, the amygdale is highly important for the process of fear conditioning, which is essential to understand social learning and offers interesting insights in human evolution. Olsson and Phelps (2007) examined amygdale activity in the context of fear conditioning and social learning. They used the fMRI method to investigate amygdale activity in reaction to conditioned stimuli (electronic shock). There are three different ways in which the amygdale is active in human beings when it comes to fear conditioning. Firstly, it shows activity in direct fear conditioning (when the test person is presented a neutral stimulus while receiving a shock). Secondly, there is amygdale activity in observed fear conditioning (when the person observes another human getting presented a stimulus and receiving a shock). Thirdly and most importantly, the amygdale is active when learning from instructed fear. This is the case when someone tells us that a certain stimulus on the screen will make us receive a shock (Olsson & Phelps, 2007). Arguably, this ability is unique to humans and may be an essential reason, why the human race carried through dangerous situations in their evolutional development.

When it comes to social interaction and regulation, empathy is a highly interesting matter. Singer (2004) shows that empathy for pain involves activation of the affective pain network, consisting of ACC and Insula, but not somatosensory areas. Based on this, concrete and highly practicable issues can be addressed. For instance, Singer et al. (2006) addressed the question if empathy depends on the behaviour of the affected person. The research team designed a study with strangers of which only one was the test person and two were confederates. The persons play an economic game called the prisoner's dilemma. One of the confederates plays fair, the other one plays unfair. Consistently, the unfair player was rated negatively, whereas the fair player got a positive rating. In a second stage, the confederates get administered an electronic shock. Measuring brain activity through fMRI, female test persons show empathy for both fair and unfair player, when they get shocked. In contrast, male test persons show less activation in ACC and Insula when the unfair player gets the pain stimulus. Additionally, the nucleus accumbens (part of the meso-limbic reward system) is activated, when the unfair player gets shocked. This activity correlates with the self-assessed 'desire for revenge' of the male proband (Singer et al., 2006). In this particular study, relevance information for neuroeconomics, evolutionary psychology and gender studies can be found. The question rises, why there is a discrepancy between men and women in felt empathy for the unfair player. It is plausible that physical punishment is more common for men. From an evolutionary perspective one could argue that punishment of norm violations was ever since rather the field of competence of men (Höhl, 2014).

Social-neuroscientific findings are not only relevant for understanding collective behaviour. They are as well of big importance for clinical aspects and aspects of individual differences in people. Especially empathy plays a fundamental role in clinical psychology, which we will investigate by taking a look at the relations of empathy and psychopathology.

Decety and Meyer (2008) formed a theoretical model of empathy for pain, postulating interactions of executive functions and emotional regulation in the prefrontal cortex (PFC), discrimination of the self and others in the parietal cortex and divided neural networks for experienced pain (activation of ACC, Insula and somatosensory areals) and pain of others (activation of ACC and Insula). People with psychopathic behaviour patterns inter alia show deficits in self-control (reactive aggression), lack of adopting social norms and significant lack of empathy and regret (Höhl, 2014). Substantiating this, psychopaths show distinct neurological conspicuities compared to unaffected people: fMRI scans of people with psychopathic personality reveal limited amygdale function and a lower skin-conductance level (indicator for stress) in fear conditioning tasks (Birbaumer et al., 2005). This explains why they lack adopting social norms. Furthermore they have problems with emotional regulation (explaining reactive aggression) and show reduced grey substance in the MPFC and temporal pole, areas necessary for mental adoption of perspectives, which verifies their problems with feeling empathy for others. As it can be seen, findings like these prove the big clinical relevance of neuroscientific research.

The last network to be addressed briefly is the mirror/simulation/action-perception network. Rizzolatti and Craighero (2004) show that mirror neurons are active in the process of learning by imitation. They postulate that observation of actions which shall be imitated activate the mirror neuron system. When the action is new to the observer, the mirror neuron system will cut it into fragments of actions that are already known, thus, activating the corresponding motoric representations. In a last step, these activated representations of the individual action fragments are merged and connected in accordance with the model action (Rizzolatti &

Craighero, 2004). Mirror neurons and there functioning are still not researched exhaustively, but they offer fascinating insights in the research area of social learning.

Having investigated findings on the social brain and having outlined their relevance for a better understanding of social interaction, the evaluation of the claim that studying brain structure and function will do little to improve our understanding of social interaction must entail a very clear denial. Of course there are potential stumbling blocks in neuroscientific argumentation (such as reverse inference) and researchers must be careful, what the explanatory potential of their methods (e.g. fMRI) is. Furthermore, promises of salvation as made in *Das Manifest* are not realistic, but it is undeniable that social neuroscience has, and will further have, a prominent role in understanding social behaviour, albeit it is clear that this requires more than neuroscience and indeed more than biology (Adolphs, 2010). Therefore, social neuroscience cannot make the claim to be the only research area that investigates social interaction the right way. On the other hand, without it, there will be no insight in underlying mechanisms of social behaviour. Social neuroscience has already contributed a lot to the understanding of individual differences in humans and collective behaviour and assuredly, there will be many more exciting findings in the future.

References

Adolphs, R. (2010). Conceptual Challenges and Directions for Social Neuroscience. *Neuron, 65*(6), 752-767. http://dx.doi.org/10.1016/j.neuron.2010.03.006

Arts, A., Anderson, C., Anderson, J., van Assen, M., Attridge, P., & Attwood, A. et al. (2016). *OSF | Reproducibility Project: Psychology*. *Osf.io*. Retrieved 18 March 2016, from https://osf.io/ezcuj/

Birbaumer, N., Veit, R., Lotze, M., Erb, M., Hermann, C., Grodd, W., & Flor, H. (2005). Deficient Fear Conditioning in Psychopathy. *Arch Gen Psychiatry, 62*(7), 799. http://dx.doi.org/10.1001/archpsyc.62.7.799

Decety, J., & Meyer, M. (2008). From emotion resonance to empathic understanding: A social developmental neuroscience account. *Develop. Psychopathol., 20*(04), 1053. http://dx.doi.org/10.1017/s0954579408000503

Dell'Amore, C. (2009). *Bikinis Make Men See Women as Objects, Scans Confirm.News.nationalgeographic.com*. Retrieved 9 March 2016, from http://news.nationalgeographic.com/news/2009/02/090216-bikinis-women-men-objects.html

Elger, E., Friederici, A., Koch, C., Luhmann, H., von der Malsburg, C., & Menzel, R. et al. (2004). *Das Manifest*. *Spektrum.de*. Retrieved 18 March 2016, from http://www.spektrum.de/thema/das-manifest/852357

Human Brain Project. (2016). *Humanbrainproject.eu*. Retrieved 21 March 2016, from https://www.humanbrainproject.eu/mission;jsessionid=j9hca47e0l7psl14akogw6se

Iacoboni, M., Freedman, J., & Kaplan, J. (2007). *This Is Your Brain on Politics*. *Nytimes.com*. Retrieved 8 March 2016, from http://www.nytimes.com/2007/11/11/opinion/11freedman.html?_r=0

Kennedy, D., & Adolphs, R. (2012). The social brain in psychiatric and neurological disorders. *Trends In Cognitive Sciences, 16*(11), 559-572. http://dx.doi.org/10.1016/j.tics.2012.09.006

Kensinger, E., & Schacter, D. (2006). Processing emotional pictures and words: Effects of valence and arousal. *Cognitive, Affective, & Behavioral Neuroscience, 6*(2), 110-126. http://dx.doi.org/10.3758/cabn.6.2.110

Lieberman, M. (2007). Social Cognitive Neuroscience: A Review of Core Processes. *Annual Review Of Psychology*, *58*(1), 259-289. http://dx.doi.org/10.1146/annurev.psych.58.110405.085654

Löken, L., Wessberg, J., Morrison, I., McGlone, F., & Olausson, H. (2009). Coding of pleasant touch by unmyelinated afferents in humans. *Nature Neuroscience*, *12*(5), 547-548. http://dx.doi.org/10.1038/nn.2312

McCabe, D., & Castel, A. (2008). Seeing is believing: The effect of brain images on judgments of scientific reasoning. *Cognition*, *107*(1), 343-352. http://dx.doi.org/10.1016/j.cognition.2007.07.017

Mitchell, J. (2006). Mentalizing and Marr: An information processing approach to the study of social cognition. *Brain Research*, *1079*(1), 66-75. http://dx.doi.org/10.1016/j.brainres.2005.12.113

Mitchell, J., Heatherton, T., & Macrae, C. (2002). Distinct neural systems subserve person and object knowledge. *Proceedings Of The National Academy Of Sciences*, *99*(23), 15238-15243. http://dx.doi.org/10.1073/pnas.232395699

Öhman, A., & Mineka, S. (2001). Fears, phobias, and preparedness: Toward an evolved module of fear and fear learning. *Psychological Review*, *108*(3), 483-522. http://dx.doi.org/10.1037/0033-295x.108.3.483

Olsson, A., & Phelps, E. (2007). Social learning of fear. *Nature Neuroscience*, *10*(9), 1095-1102. http://dx.doi.org/10.1038/nn1968

Rizzolatti, G., & Craighero, L. (2004). THE MIRROR-NEURON SYSTEM. *Annu. Rev. Neurosci.*, *27*(1), 169-192. http://dx.doi.org/10.1146/annurev.neuro.27.070203.144230

Schmundt, H., & Felix, H. (2012). *Kritik an Neuroscans: "Hirnforscher sollten nicht überreizen" - SPIEGEL ONLINE*. *SPIEGEL ONLINE*. Retrieved 21 March 2016, from http://www.spiegel.de/wissenschaft/mensch/kritik-an-fmrt-hirnscans-interview-mit-felix-hasler-a-867591.html

Singer, T. (2004). Empathy for Pain Involves the Affective but not Sensory Components of Pain. *Science*, *303*(5661), 1157-1162. http://dx.doi.org/10.1126/science.1093535

Singer, T., Seymour, B., O'Doherty, J., Stephan, K., Dolan, R., & Frith, C. (2006). Empathic neural responses are modulated by the perceived fairness of others. *Nature*, *439*(7075), 466-469. http://dx.doi.org/10.1038/nature04271

Wager, T., Lindquist, M., & Kaplan, L. (2007). Meta-analysis of functional neuroimaging data: current and future directions. *Social Cognitive And Affective Neuroscience*, *2*(2), 150-158. http://dx.doi.org/10.1093/scan/nsm01

YOUR KNOWLEDGE HAS VALUE

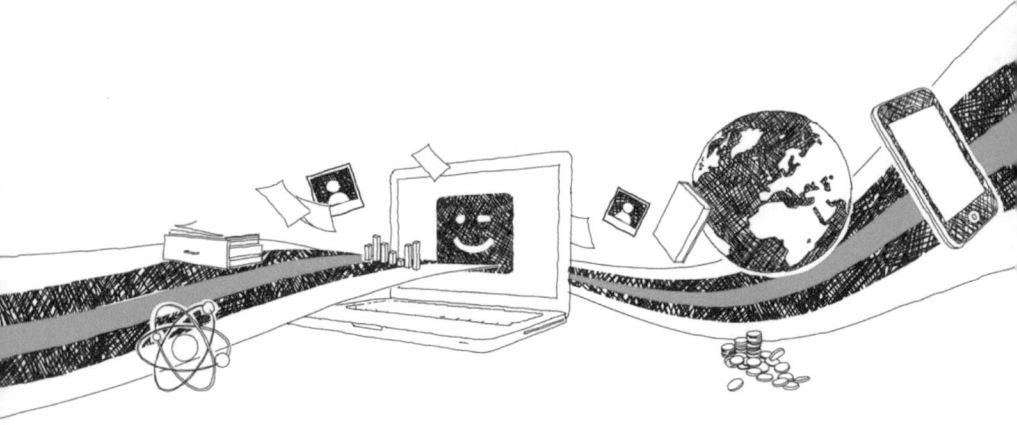

- We will publish your bachelor's and master's thesis, essays and papers

- Your own eBook and book - sold worldwide in all relevant shops

- Earn money with each sale

Upload your text at www.GRIN.com
and publish for free

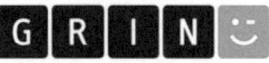